COLOUR GUIDE

Imaging

D. N. Redhead MB ChB DMRD FRCR

Consultant Radiologist, The Royal Infirmary of Edinburgh,
Edinburgh, UK

Churchill Livingstone

EDINBURGH LONDON MADRID MELBOURNE NEW YORK AND TOKYO 1995

CHURCHILL LIVINGSTONE
Medical Division of Pearson Professional Limited

Distributed in the United States of America by
Churchill Livingstone Inc., 650 Avenue of the Americas,
New York, N.Y. 10011, and by associated companies,
branches and representatives throughout the world.

© Pearson Professional Limited 1995

First published 1995

ISBN 0–443–05020–1

British Library Cataloguing in Publication Data
A catalogue record for this book is available from the
British Library.

Library of Congress Cataloging in Publication Data
A catalogue record for this book is available from the
Library of Congress.

*For Churchill
Livingstone*

Publisher
Laurence Hunter
Project Editor
Jim Killgore
Production
Nancy Arnott
Kay Hunston
Design Direction
Erik Bigland
Sales Promotion Executive
Duncan Jones

Printed in Hong Kong
GC/01

Preface

Radiological imaging, combining art and science, is particularly suitable for inclusion in the Colour Guide series. The ever increasing array of sophisticated technologies provides explicit, detailed and sometimes coloured displays of human anatomy, its anomalies and its abnormalities. The choice of tests, the order in which they should be applied and the expanding selection of therapeutic interventional procedures presents for the initiated, as well as for the uninitiated, a fascinating but sometimes confusing picture. It is hoped that this text will provide, at the turn of a page, an easy guide to radiological investigation and management. Where the investigative pathways are complex, algorithms have been provided. Illustrations have been chosen to display classical and relevant features in many common clinical situations.

I would like to acknowledge the assistance of Dr Nicholas Chalmers and the many colleagues who have generously contributed illustrations for the book. I am especially indebted to Dr Ian Beggs, Dr Robin Sellar, Dr Irene Prossor, Dr John Reid, Dr Nicé Muir, Dr Ian Gillespie, Dr Andrew Wright and Dr Donald Collie. I would also take this opportunity to thank the Medical Illustration Department at Edinburgh University for their patience and care in preparing the illustrations, and also to thank Linda McVicar and Gillian Clement for their assistance in the preparation of the manuscript.

1995   D.N.R.

Contents

YEŞNE ALICI

1 / Diagnostic imaging modalities

X-rays

Basic principles   X-rays are short-wavelength electromagnetic radiation. They are produced when high velocity electrons, accelerated across an evacuated tube at high voltage, hit a tungsten anode (Fig. 1). The X-ray beam emerges from the tube through a window in a lead shield. X-ray photons interact with matter in several ways. For practical purposes, they pass relatively unimpeded through materials of low density and low atomic weight, but a higher proportion of photons are stopped by dense substances and particularly by elements of high atomic weight. Hence the ability of lead to provide protection. When X-ray photons hit a phosphor screen light is emitted, which can be detected by photographic film or amplified by an image intensifier to produce a visible image in real time (fluoroscopy). Modern radiological equipment involves highly sophisticated and complex technology (Fig. 2).

Risks   The benefits to patients of diagnostic radiation greatly outweigh the risks. However, the dangers of radiation must not be ignored and the doses patients receive must be as low as is compatible with good patient care. The most significant risk is carcinogenesis. The risk of fatal cancer is estimated at 0.005% per mSv (milliSievert) for all ages, and 0.01% per mSv for the fetus. Most examinations deliver doses in the range 0.1–10 mSv. Computed tomography (CT) produces high patient doses.

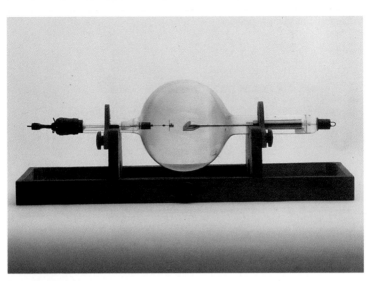

Fig. 1 X-ray tube.

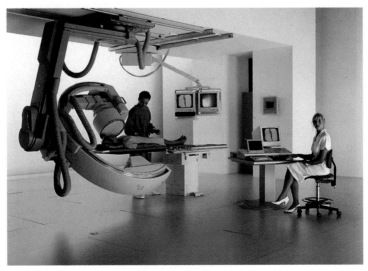

Fig. 2 Modern angiography suite. (Courtesy of Philips Medical)

Conventional radiology

Basic principles Gas, fat and water can be differentiated on a radiograph due to differences in density. Soft tissue has similar characteristics to water. Bone causes much higher X-ray absorption because of the high atomic weight of calcium so can be readily detected. Radiographic diagnosis depends on the analysis of the pattern of these densities (Fig. 3). Iodine and barium are atoms of high atomic weight and have appropriate chemical properties which allow their use as contrast media.

Digital imaging

Basic principles Computer techniques permit significant advances in image manipulation and storage. The radiographic image is first digitised, i.e. divided into a matrix of small squares or pixels. Each pixel is assigned a numerical value according to its radiographic density. Digital technology allows lower doses of radiation than does conventional radiography.

Applications Digital subtraction involves acquiring an image prior to, and during, administration of contrast medium. The value of each pixel in the first image is then subtracted from the second, resulting in an image showing only the added contrast medium. This is particularly useful in angiography (Fig. 4), allowing smaller contrast volumes to be used.

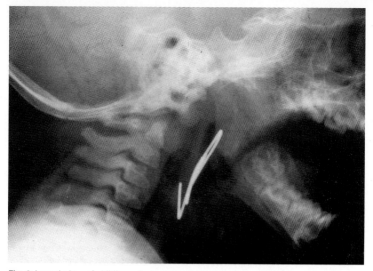

Fig. 3 Lateral view of child's neck showing air, bone, metal and soft tissue densities. The paperclip has perforated the pharynx.

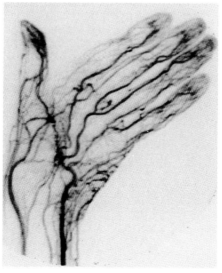

Fig. 4 Digital angiogram of arteries of the hand.

Computed tomography (CT)

Basic principles In CT, the X-ray tube is rotated around the patient and the X-ray beam impinges on an array of detectors as it emerges from the patient. The intensity of the transmitted beam at each angle is recorded. By a computer technique involving the solution of many simultaneous equations, a two-dimensional image is produced of an axial slice through the patient. The value of each pixel depends on the attenuation of the X-ray beam by the small volume of the tissue that the pixel represents. As with conventional radiography, there is differential attenuation of the beam by tissues of different atomic weight and density. With CT, very small differences in attenuation can be detected, allowing differentiation of cerebral grey and white matter, for example (Figs 5, 6).

The Hounsfield scale is used, by convention, as a measure of radiation attenuation of the tissues in CT. Water has a value of 0, soft tissues are usually in the range 20 to 60, whereas calcium is over 100. Fat is in the range −40 to −80 (Fig. 7), and air is −1000.

Applications The advent of CT revolutionised diagnostic imaging of the central nervous system by allowing noninvasive imaging of intracranial structures. It has subsequently found many further applications, especially in the mediastinum and retroperitoneum.

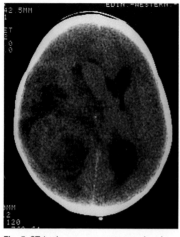

Fig. 5 CT brain scan, precontrast, showing malignant glioma.

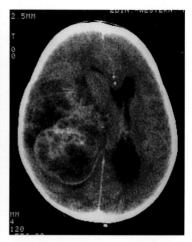

Fig. 6 CT brain scan of same patient, post-contrast, showing tumour enhancement.

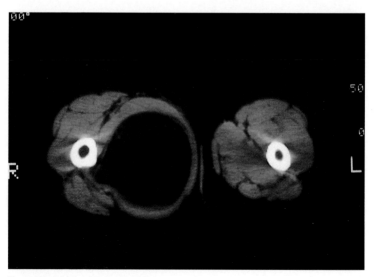

Fig. 7 CT of thigh, showing large lipoma.

Ultrasound

Basic principles When high-frequency sound waves pass through soft tissues, echoes are produced at interfaces, such as the renal capsule or the bile duct wall. Knowing the speed of sound in soft tissues, the depth of the source of the echo can be calculated from the time lapse between production of the sound and detection of the echo. This one-dimensional information is the basis of M-mode ultrasound, which is useful for studying movement of the heart valves. When an ultrasound beam is scanned through an arc, combining the direction of the beam with the depth of the echo allows a two-dimensional image to be produced (B-mode). Modern ultrasound machines permit rapid scanning, resulting in a 'real-time' image. The ultrasound beam cannot penetrate bone or air. This restricts the use of ultrasound to soft tissues.

Applications Since fluid provides an ultrasound 'window', the fetus is well seen in the amniotic sac. Ultrasound is the imaging modality of choice in the field of obstetrics.

It is the initial modality used in the assessment of patients with hepatobiliary (Fig. 8), pancreatic, renal or gynaecological symptoms. It is valuable in the detection of fluid collections and abscesses, and can be employed to guide aspiration or drainage manoeuvres.

Doppler

Basic principles When sound waves are echoed from a moving object, e.g. flowing blood cells, the frequency alters. The frequency shift depends on both the velocity and on the direction of movement in relation to the beam. A focal stenosis in an artery produces a high velocity jet, whereas an occluded vessel produces no Doppler signal.

Applications Doppler is increasingly used to evaluate the patient with arterial problems, particularly those with lower limb or carotid disease. Ultrasound with Doppler imaging can also be used in the evaluation of the venous system (Fig. 9).

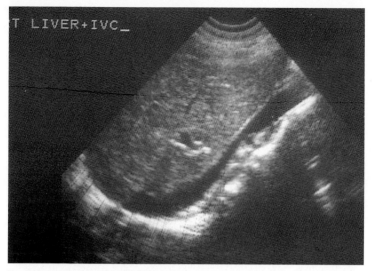

Fig. 8 Ultrasound of liver, normal examination.

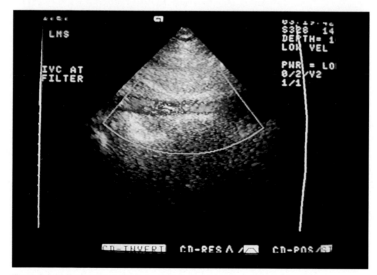

Fig. 9 Colour Doppler examination of inferior vena cava showing normal flow.

Nuclear medicine

Basic principles   The radioisotopes used in nuclear medicine imaging produce gamma rays. Apart from their source, gamma rays are identical to X-rays. The gamma camera consists of a collimator, a phosphor screen and an array of photomultiplier tubes connected to a computer. Gamma rays are emitted from the patient in all directions. This would result in a blurred image so a collimator is required. This absorbs all photons except those emanating from tissues directly perpendicular to it, resulting in a sharp image on the screen. The image differs from a radiograph in that it reflects function rather than structure alone (Fig. 10).

Applications   By selecting a radiopharmaceutical with appropriate properties, a range of organs (Figs 11, 12) and functions can be examined. Technetium-99m (^{99m}Tc) is used for most examinations. It produces only gamma rays — no harmful alpha or beta particles. It has a half-life of 6 hours, allowing time for the image acquisition but decaying to negligible levels in a day or two. It is readily obtainable from a portable molybdenum generator and, being a transitional element, can be easily bound to a range of organic compounds with appropriate pharmacological properties.

^{99m}Tc-labelled hepatoiminodiacetic acid (^{99m}Tc/HIDA) is useful in hepatobiliary imaging as its secretion is similar to that of bile.

For perfusion lung scanning, the isotope ^{99m}Tc-labelled macroaggregated albumin is used. The small particles labelled with the isotope demonstrate pulmonary blood flow.

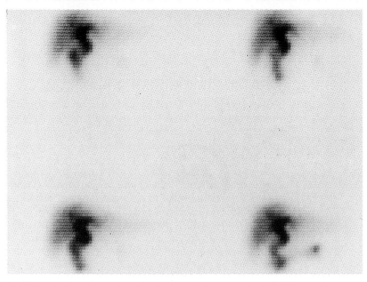

Fig. 10 Isotope liver scan demonstrating normal isotope excretion in biliary system.

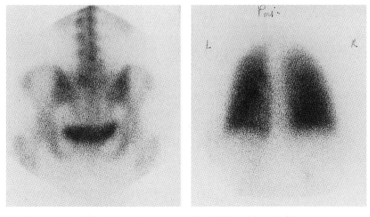

Fig. 11 Normal isotope bone scan.

Fig. 12 Normal isotope lung scan.

Magnetic resonance imaging (MRI)

Basic principles The principles of MRI are complicated. Hydrogen nuclei (protons) have a magnetic dipole so that they line up in a strong magnetic field. When exposed to a radio-wave pulse at a certain resonant frequency, they are knocked out of line. The resonant frequency (Larmor frequency) depends on the magnetic field strength. When the radio-pulse is switched off, the protons 'precess' back to the resting state, releasing energy in the form of a radio-frequency signal. In MRI (Fig. 13), the patient is placed in a powerful magnet and exposed to a series of radio-pulses. Radio-signals emitted by the protons in the patient are detected by receiver coils. These signals give rise to the image. Spatial information is derived by applying magnetic field gradients across the patient. Thus, only those protons in the slice at the appropriate field strength will resonate in response to the radio pulse. The intensity and duration of the signal emitted depend on the density of hydrogen nuclei and the degree to which they are bound in the tissues. Differences in these parameters provide soft tissue contrast.

Applications MRI is of great value in the brain (Fig. 14), spine and joints. Its role in the thorax and abdomen (Fig. 15) is not yet established.

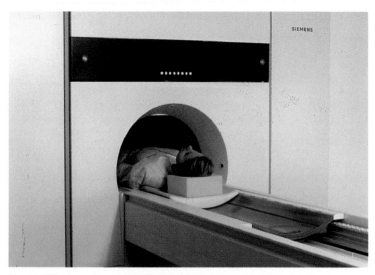

Fig. 13 MRI scanner (Courtesy of Siemens Medical)

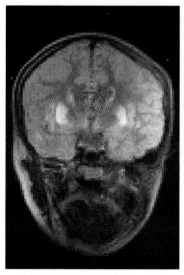

Fig. 14 MRI examination of the brain.

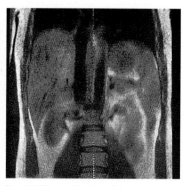

Fig. 15 MRI examination of the abdomen.

Interventional radiology

Basic principles

This subspecialty is concerned with a range of percutaneous therapeutic procedures which are performed using diagnostic imaging techniques for guidance. It can be conveniently divided into vascular and nonvascular procedures. However, the principles of access, imaging guidance and guide-wire/catheter manipulation apply to both.

Access to the target organ or vessel usually involves the Seldinger technique. A needle is introduced percutaneously, and a guide-wire is passed through the needle into the vessel or organ. The needle is removed and the percutaneous tract dilated as required to permit passage of a catheter over the wire. This technique allows safe and relatively atraumatic access.

Imaging guidance is generally by fluoroscopy or by ultrasound. Where the target structure is not seen well on ultrasound, CT may be used to guide the needle puncture accurately.

Applications

In general, most vascular interventional procedures are performed under fluoroscopic guidance. They include angioplasty, where a narrowed vessel is dilated using a balloon catheter (Fig. 16), or stenting, where the patency of a vessel is maintained by insertion of a wire-mesh tube or stent.

Nonvascular interventions include drainage procedures, in which a large-bore, multiple-holed tube is introduced to decompress or drain an obstructed system, such as the urinary system (nephrostomy), or an abscess or fluid collection.

Having achieved access to a specific area, further more complex manoeuvres can be performed. In the urinary tract or biliary system, for example, stones can be removed using a stone-catching basket (Fig. 17). Stents may be used to maintain patency in other situations, e.g. where a pancreatic carcinoma has caused a biliary stricture or to support the liver tract of a portosystemic shunt (Figs 18, 19).

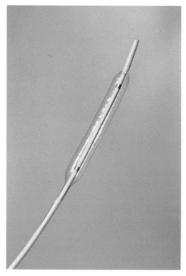

Fig. 16 Balloon catheter.

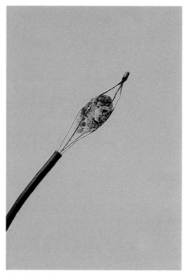

Fig. 17 Basket used for percutaneous biliary or ureteric stone extraction.

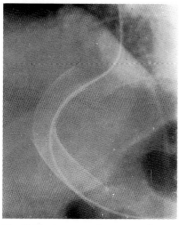

Fig. 18 Metal stent used to support liver shunt.

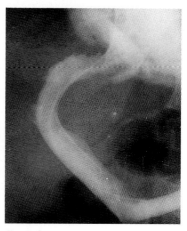

Fig. 19 Contrast demonstrating good flow through shunt.

2 / Cardiovascular imaging

Conventional radiology

An examination of the cardiac size and contour can provide valuable information in patients with cardiac problems. Normally, the cardiac size is less than 50% of the maximum diameter of the thorax (Fig. 20). In left ventricular failure the heart is enlarged. There may be other signs of elevated pulmonary venous pressure. These are, progressively: distension of the upper lobe veins, horizontal pleural-based lines in the lower zones (Kerley B lines) caused by fluid in the interlobular septae, and fluffy, ill-defined pulmonary shadowing due to alveolar pulmonary oedema.

Causes of left ventricular failure include myocardial infarction and aortic valve disease. In aortic stenosis, calcification may be seen in relation to the valve. Dilatation of the aortic root may also be a feature.

Alterations in cardiac contour may also provide a clue to diagnosis. For example, in mitral valve disease, particularly regurgitation, the left atrium appears enlarged (Fig. 21). This causes a characteristic double right cardiac border, splaying of the carina, and a hump on the upper left cardiac border caused by a distended left atrial appendage.

With tricuspid valve disease, the cardiac chambers on the right side of the heart may show enlargement. Some forms of congenital heart disease produce characteristic cardiac contours; for example, with Fallot's tetralogy the contour has been described as 'boot-shaped', and complete transposition like a 'snowman'.

Ultrasound

Echocardiography (cardiac ultrasound) can be performed with a transducer on the chest wall or in the oesophagus. It shows chamber size, myocardial thickness and motion. Valve motion is assessed by M-mode and real-time, whereas stenotic or regurgitant jets are demonstrated by Doppler ultrasound.

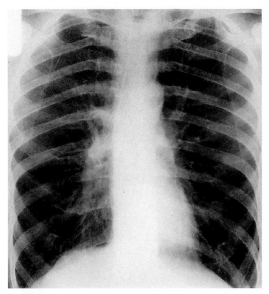

Fig. 20 Normal chest X-ray.

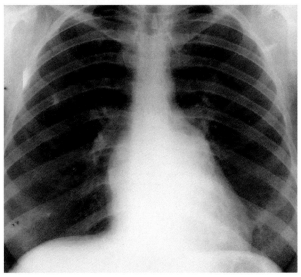

Fig. 21 Chest film showing features of mitral stenosis.

Nuclear medicine

Ventriculography
Myocardial function can be assessed by the use of ^{99m}Tc-labelled red cells. Images are acquired with ECG gating so that the image of each phase of the cardiac cycle is summed over many cycles. From the number of counts in the end-systole and the end-diastole images, the ejection fraction is calculated. This is the proportion of the end-diastolic volume ejected during systole, normally 50–70%.
A normal left ventricle contracts uniformly; infarcted muscle shows impaired or paradoxical motion.

Thallium scanning
The distribution of thallium when injected intravenously reflects myocardial bloodflow. During exercise there is diminished uptake in areas of ischaemia as compared with normal myocardium (Fig. 22). After a rest, thallium is washed out of normal areas more quickly so there is an apparent filling in of the ischaemic regions (Fig. 23). Infarcts do not take up thallium and so do not 'fill in' on the delayed scan.

^{99m}Tc-pyrophosphate scanning
^{99m}Tc-pyrophosphate binds to calcium in infarcted, but not in normal, myocardium. This can be useful in confirming the presence and location of an infarct if cardiac enzymes and ECG are equivocal. The peak uptake is 48–72 hours after infarction.

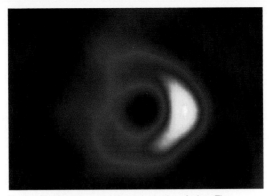

Fig. 22 Thallium scan showing impaired perfusion. The doughnut shape should be complete.

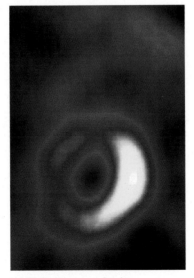

Fig. 23 Thallium scan showing improvement after a rest period.

Angiography

Left heart catheterisation

A catheter is introduced using the Seldinger technique into the femoral artery, and advanced up the aorta and across the aortic valve. Contrast is injected during rapid filming. Ventricular wall motion, ejection fraction, mitral regurgitation and aortic stenosis (Fig. 24) can be assessed. The pressure gradient across the aortic valve indicates the severity of the stenosis.

Coronary angiography

Contrast is injected into each coronary artery (Fig. 25). Stenoses (Fig. 26) or occlusions are demonstrated. Some are treated by balloon dilatation (angioplasty). The risks of angioplasty include dissection, which requires emergency bypass surgery in 4–5%. Recurrence of stenosis occurs in 40%.

Right heart catheterisation

This method permits assessment of valve dysfunction. Introducing a catheter from the femoral vein, pressure measurements are taken in the right atrium, right ventricle and pulmonary artery. The catheter tip can be wedged in a pulmonary artery; the wedge pressure is equal to the left atrial pressure. Simultaneous measurement of left ventricular end-diastolic and wedge pressure gives the gradient across the mitral valve and thus the severity of mitral stenosis.

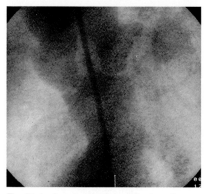

Fig. 24 Angiogram showing aortic stenosis.

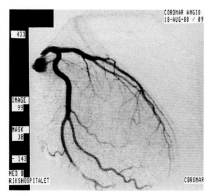

Fig. 25 Normal coronary angiogram.

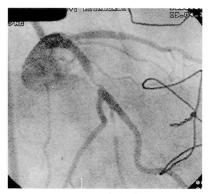

Fig. 26 Coronary artery stenosis.

Arteries

Angiography

Angiography (Fig. 27) is currently the primary means of demonstration of arterial disease affecting the lower limbs. Percutaneous catheterisation of the femoral artery is performed and a catheter placed in the abdominal aorta. Contrast is introduced and a series of films obtained as the contrast column passes through the arterial system to the feet. A conventional or digital substraction technique may be used.

Angiography will demonstrate stenoses or occlusions (Fig. 28) in the arterial system. The distribution of disease determines the most appropriate therapy. Long chronic occlusions are best treated by surgical bypass, and acute embolism causing neurosensory deficit requires emergency surgical embolectomy. Increasingly, however, less severe forms of peripheral arterial disease are treated by radiological intervention.

Interventional radiology

Percutaneous transluminal angioplasty (PTA). This is used for the treatment of stenoses or short occlusions (Figs 29, 30). It is most successful in iliac stenoses, with around 60% patency after 5 years. Results are less good in complete occlusions and in more peripheral arteries.

Thrombolysis. This is used in the management of acute and subacute arterial occlusion. A catheter is embedded in the clot, and low-dose plasminogen activator, urokinase or streptokinase is infused over several hours. Any underlying stenosis may be treated by angioplasty.

Stents. These are wire-mesh cylinders used to maintain patency, especially where angioplasty fails.

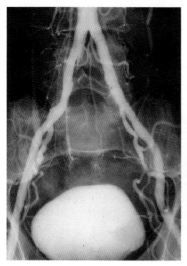

Fig. 27 Aorto-iliac angiogram.

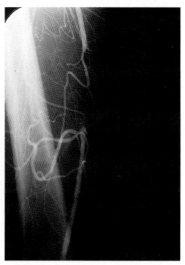

Fig. 28 Short occlusion of superficial femoral artery.

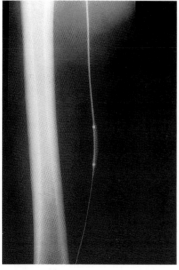

Fig. 29 Recanalisation of occluded segment.

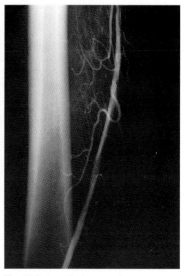

Fig. 30 Post-angioplasty result.

Doppler
ultrasound This is becoming increasingly important in the investigation of arterial disease, particularly in the extracranial carotid arteries (Figs 31, 32) and in the lower limbs.

In general, a stenosis of 50%-diameter reduction does not produce haemodynamic changes. When the diameter reduction exceeds 50% there is an increase in flow velocity through the lesion which is roughly proportional to the severity of the stenosis. When the stenosis is extreme there is a reduction in flow velocity. No flow signal is obtained from a complete occlusion.

MRI Magnetic resonance imaging is valuable in the evaluation of a number of cardiovascular disorders. In the heart it can provide an assessment of structure and function. It can demonstrate chamber volume and, in addition, can give functional information regarding the myocardial wall and the valves.

The clear depiction of vascular structures on MRI has been hampered by motion artefact. However, technological developments in this field now permit acceptable demonstration of certain areas. Currently the main applications are in the extracranial carotid arteries and in the cerebral circulation. This modality is not generally available at the present time.

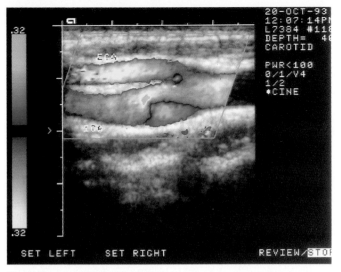

Fig. 31 Normal carotid Doppler study.

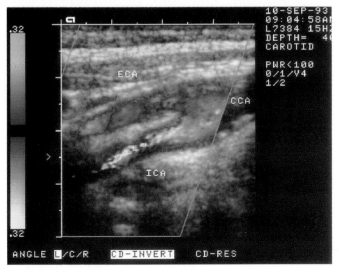

Fig. 32 Carotid artery stenosis.

Aortic imaging

Traumatic rupture of the thoracic aorta

CT and angiography

This is not uncommon following high-speed road accidents. The chest X-ray is nonspecific, showing widening of the mediastinum (Fig. 33). CT is sensitive in the detection of a peri-aortic haematoma, and this finding is an indication for thoracic aortography. A false aneurysm or an intimal flap may be seen, most commonly just beyond the origin of the left subclavian artery. Spontaneous aortic dissection (Fig. 34) gives similar nonspecific findings on the plain radiograph. The extent of the dissection is important in determining management.

Abdominal aortic aneurysm

Ultrasound and CT

Ultrasound is the simplest investigation of abdominal aortic aneurysm. Aneurysm diameter is important in determining the risk/benefit ratio of elective surgery. Angiography provides a road map to guide elective repair. Where rupture is suspected and the presentation is typical, imaging is not required. If the diagnosis is in doubt, CT is the most appropriate investigation (Fig. 35).

Interventional radiology

The development of 'covered' stents, i.e. wire-mesh tubes which have a fabric covering, has stimulated interest in their use in the management of aortic aneurysms. It is likely that in the future some aortic aneurysms will be managed by percutaneous introduction of covered stents.

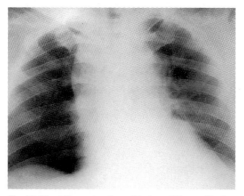

Fig. 33 Chest X-ray showing widening of the mediastinum.

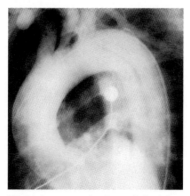

Fig. 34 Aortogram showing an intimal flap in thoracic dissection.

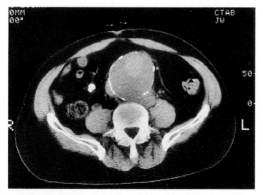

Fig. 35 CT showing abdominal aortic aneurysm.

Veins: deep venous thrombosis (Fig. 36)

Contrast studies

Venography. This involves the injection of contrast into a vein on the dorsum of the foot, with tourniquets above the ankle and knee to occlude the superficial veins. Thrombus is identified as a filling defect (Fig. 37). Films of the deep veins from the ankles to the inferior vena cava are obtained.

Ultrasound

A less invasive test which avoids the risk of radiation (important in the pregnant patient), can reliably identify clot in the femoropopliteal segment, but is less accurate in evaluating calf or pelvic vein clot.

Interventional radiology

Caval filter. Most pulmonary emboli arise from thrombus in the deep veins of the legs, particularly from the veins of the thigh and pelvis. Where a patient is at particular risk of pulmonary embolus, for example where there is a long segment of free floating thrombus extending from the popliteal vein to the inferior vena cava (Fig. 37) and where anticoagulation is contraindicated, the percutaneous insertion of an open mesh umbrella-like device, a caval filter (Fig. 38) can be used to prevent life-threatening clot moving to the pulmonary circulation, while at the same time preserving the patency of the cava.

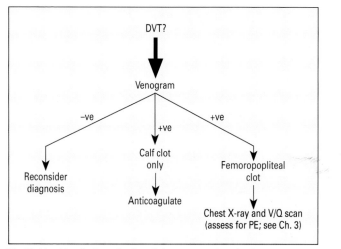

Fig. 36 Algorithm for investigation of deep venous thrombosis.

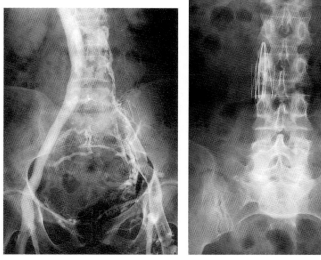

Fig. 37 High segment thrombus.

Fig. 38 Caval filter.

3 / Respiratory imaging

Anatomical landmarks

Conventional radiology

Maximising the information contained on a chest film requires a systematic check of the basic anatomical landmarks. The tracheal transradiancy should be central. The cardiac shadow should be one-third to the right of the spine, and two-thirds to the left. The hilar shadows should be of equal density and size. The lung fields should be of equal transradiancy. The diaphragmatic outline, and the costophrenic and cardiophrenic angles should be clear. The bony thoracic cage and soft tissues need to be carefully examined (see Fig. 20).

Infection

Pneumonia

Conventional radiology

In pneumonia, the alveoli or distal airspaces lose their transradiancy, being full of mucus and pus, showing either patchy or confluent consolidation (Fig. 39). The bronchi are not involved and are therefore outlined, giving an 'air bronchogram'. A pleural effusion may develop. Abscess formation (Fig. 40) may be a feature of bacterial pneumonias, such as those due to *Staphylococcus aureus*, *Klebsiella* or mycobacterium tuberculosis (TB). In this situation, a discrete round shadow often containing an air/fluid level may be seen.

Pneumocystis carinii (Fig. 41) or tuberculous pneumonia may occur as a complication of HIV infection.

Pulmonary tuberculosis

Conventional radiology

Primary TB may present with enlarged lymph nodes (Fig. 42) around the hila or paratracheal regions, with or without consolidation. A miliary pattern may be seen in post-primary TB. There is consolidation and/or cavitation, frequently at the lung apices. Scarring with bronchiectasis may result.

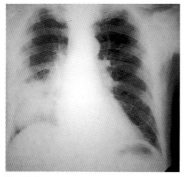

Fig. 39 Pneumonia affecting right lower lobe.

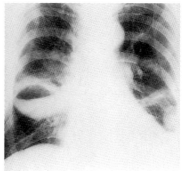

Fig. 40 Lung abscess.

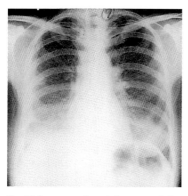

Fig. 41 Pneumocystis carinii pneumonia in an AIDS patient.

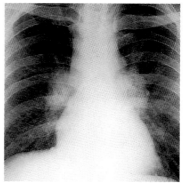

Fig. 42 Lymphadenopathy in tuberculosis.

Benign tumours

Conventional radiology

Benign lung tumours are rare and include granulomas and hamartomas (Fig. 43). They tend to be round, well defined and slow growing. Many contain calcification.

Malignant tumours

Conventional radiology

Lung cancer is the commonest malignancy in men. A mass may be seen on the chest X-ray (Fig. 44). A centrally placed lesion may lead to partial or total collapse of a lung. Secondary pneumonia is a common feature. A pleural effusion may be present. Enlarged lymph nodes in the hilar or paratracheal regions may be evident, and destruction of adjacent bony structures, such as ribs or vertebral bodies, may be seen.

Metastatic disease (Fig. 45) is suggested by the presence of multiple lesions.

CT

CT is useful in the staging of lung tumours. Solid lesions can be differentiated from vascular structures when an intravenous contrast injection is given.

MRI

MRI can also differentiate solid lesions from vascular structures, and since chronic fibrosis gives a different signal on MRI, the latter can distinguish fibrotic from neoplastic tissue.

Interventional radiology

Where proof of malignancy is necessary, this can be obtained by needle biopsy of the lesion carried out under local anaesthesia using either CT or fluoroscopic guidance. In a few patients, a small pneumothorax or haemothorax may occur as a result of this procedure.

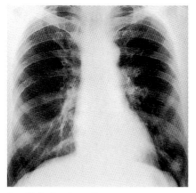

Fig. 43 Benign hamartoma.

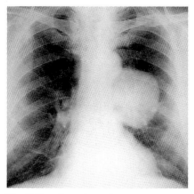

Fig. 44 Bronchogenic carcinoma.

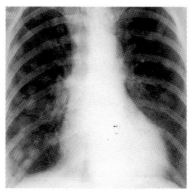

Fig. 45 Multiple intrapulmonary metastases.

Thromboembolic disease (Fig. 46)

Pulmonary emboli occur when thrombus from the lower limb or pelvic veins moves to the pulmonary circulation.

Conventional radiology

The chest X-ray may be normal, or there may be nonspecific changes such as consolidation, atelectasis or pleural effusion.

V/Q scan

The V/Q scan involves two parts, a ventilation study in which the patient inhales ^{133}Xe, and a perfusion study in which an intravenous injection of ^{99m}Tc-labelled microspheres of albumin is given. The microspheres become trapped in the pulmonary microcirculation, reflecting the pulmonary bloodflow (Fig. 47). A normal perfusion scan excludes a pulmonary embolus.

The V/Q scan is reported in conjunction with the chest X-ray, and the result given in terms of 'probability'. Where there is an abnormality such as consolidation on the chest film and where there is a corresponding defect on the perfusion scan, a report of 'low probability' of pulmonary embolus is given. On the other hand, where the lung scan and the ventilation scan are normal but the perfusion scan shows multiple defects, a diagnosis of 'high probability' of pulmonary emboli is made. In many instances the picture is not clear cut. There may be multiple perfusion defects, some matching changes on the chest X-ray or ventilation scan and one not matching. The patient may have chronic lung changes and perhaps previous pulmonary emboli. Where there is doubt regarding the diagnosis, a pulmonary angiogram is advisable.

Pulmonary angiography

Pulmonary angiography involves introducing a catheter into the femoral vein using the Seldinger technique, and passing the catheter under fluoroscopic guidance into the main pulmonary artery or selectively into the right and left pulmonary arteries in turn. Contrast is injected and films obtained. Thrombus is identified as a filling defect or as an occlusion of a branch artery (Fig. 48).

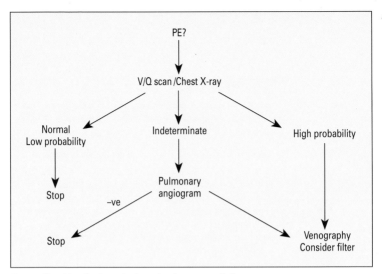

Fig. 46 Algorithm for investigation of pulmonary embolus.

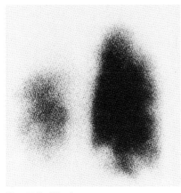

Fig. 47 Positive lung scan.

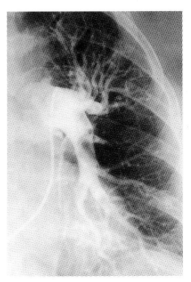

Fig. 48 Positive pulmonary angiogram.

Chest trauma

Conventional radiology

Traumatic chest injuries are generally the result of road traffic accidents. Plain X-rays allow initial assessment of the bony thoracic cage, pulmonary and vascular structures. Rib fractures (Fig. 49) may be single or multiple. If several ribs are broken in two places, a 'flail segment' will be present. Rib fractures may be associated with damage to the underlying lung and pleura, resulting in air leaking into the pleural cavity (pneumothorax) or blood collecting around the lung (haemothorax). When a pneumothorax is present, the lung edge can be clearly seen, displaced away from the ribs. If the amount of air is large, the mediastinal structures can be displaced towards the contralateral side. This constitutes an emergency and is termed a 'tension pneumothorax' (Fig. 50). Urgent intercostal drainage is required. Lung contusion gives rise to consolidation; total lung collapse with loss of lung volume, mediastinal shift and loss of aeration suggests a bronchial rupture.

Fractures involving the upper ribs raise the possibility of damage to underlying vascular structures. Fractures of lower left ribs may be associated with damage to the spleen or left kidney. The left diaphragm may be ruptured with herniation of abdominal contents into the chest. In addition to loss of the normal diaphragmatic outline, unusual gas shadows may be evident within the thoracic cavity.

Fractures of the lower right ribs may be associated with hepatic injury. Rupture of the right diaphragm is less common than on the left side.

Contrast studies

Contrast studies may be useful in confirming the position of intestinal loops.

CT and angiography

CT scanning is valuable in the assessment of the patient who has sustained chest trauma. It can detect mediastinal haemorrhage, which may reflect major vascular injury, and angiography is indicated (Fig. 51). CT may also demonstrate skeletal injuries undetected by plain films. An evaluation of the intra-abdominal structures can also be made.

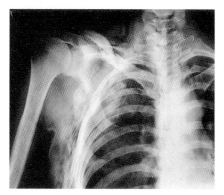

Fig. 49 Multiple rib fractures.

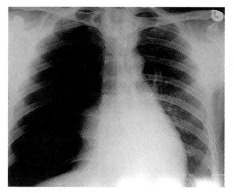

Fig. 50 Tension pneumothorax.

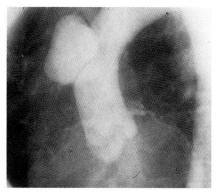

Fig. 51 Post-traumatic aneurysm of ascending aorta.

4 / Gastrointestinal imaging

Abdominal pain

Conventional radiology

Acute abdominal pain. Supine and erect abdominal films, together with an erect chest film, are valuable in the initial assessment of the patient with acute abdominal pain where intestinal obstruction or perforation is suspected. Intestinal gas provides a natural contrast allowing identification, localisation and measurement of bowel loops. Mechanical obstruction generally leads to bowel dilatation and, in the erect film, fluid-levels are observed (Fig. 52).

Free intra-abdominal gas usually indicates perforation and the most common explanation is perforation of a duodenal ulcer. The erect chest film is frequently the best film to show free gas under the diaphragm (Fig. 53).

Non-acute abdominal pain. Where abdominal pain is subacute, intermittent or chronic, a supine abdominal film may provide a clue to the diagnosis. In addition to the natural contrast medium, air, which will be seen within bowel loops, an added natural contrast, calcium may be evident. Arterial calcification is common in the older age group and in diabetics at a younger age. It may be seen within the wall of an abdominal aortic aneurysm. 15% of gallstones and 80% of renal calculi calcify. In some situations, a specific diagnosis can be made on the plain films, whereas in others the findings are nonspecific but may help in directing further investigations.

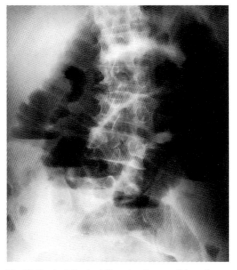

Fig. 52 Erect abdominal film showing small bowel obstruction.

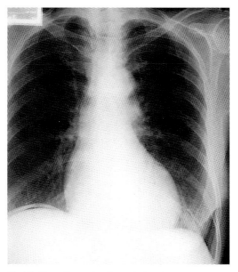

Fig. 53 Chest X-ray showing subphrenic gas.

The oesophagus

Contrast studies The routine radiological investigation of the oesophagus involves a barium study — a *barium swallow*. The barium coats the mucosa. An effervescent agent is often given in addition; this distends the oesophagus. The combination of barium and air provides two different contrast agents, giving a 'double contrast' study. The oesophageal mucosa is clearly demonstrated (Fig. 54), and information relating to oesophageal motility is also provided.

The barium swallow readily allows demonstration of common problems, including hiatus hernia (Fig. 55), webs (Fig. 56), inflammatory changes and strictures. Differentiation between benign and malignant strictures can be difficult. Benign strictures have a tapering appearance while malignant lesions tend to have a shouldered margin (Fig. 57).

Ultrasound There is an increasing interest in the use of endoscopic ultrasound in the evaluation of intramural lesions. This technique involves introducing an endoscope incorporating an ultrasound facility into the oesophagus. This allows direct visualisation of a lesion involving the oesophageal mucosa and an evaluation of the extra-oesophageal component.

Endoscopic ultrasound is not generally available at the present time.

CT An assessment of resectability of an oesophageal lesion is more usually made by using CT scanning. Like endoscopic ultrasound, it can assess the extra-oesophageal component of the lesion and detect invasion of adjacent structures and enlargement of draining lymph nodes.

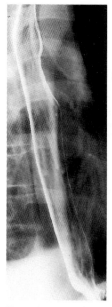

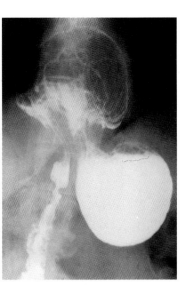

Fig. 54 Normal barium swallow.

Fig. 55 Large hiatus hernia.

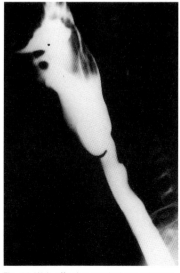

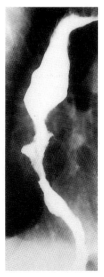

Fig. 56 Web affecting cervical oesophagus.

Fig. 57 Extensive oesophageal carcinoma.

Stomach and duodenum

Contrast studies

The double-contrast barium study of the stomach and duodenum — the *barium meal* — requires a meticulous technique and multiple views to obtain optimal results. As with the barium swallow technique, the patient ingests a cupful of barium to coat the mucosa, and an effervecent agent to distend the stomach and duodenum. Some radiologists routinely administer the antispasmodic drug, Buscopan (hyoscine-N-butylbromide) to abolish spasm and peristalsis during the procedure.

Benign ulcers. Most *gastric ulcers* are located on the lesser curve (Fig. 58) or the posterior wall of the stomach, while most *duodenal ulcers* affect the anterior wall (Fig. 60). Barium collects in the ulcer crater. Mucosal folds can be seen radiating to the crater. Benign gastric ulcers tend to project outside the lumen of the stomach. However, many benign ulcers do not show typical features and endoscopy with biopsy confirmation is advisable. A small percentage of duodenal ulcers occur in the postbulbar region. Where there are multiple ulcers and thickening of the mucosal folds, the Zollinger-Ellison syndrome, due to a gastrin-secreting non-beta islet cell tumour, should be considered.

Malignant ulcers have a nodular pattern outside the ulcer crater and the folds do not reach the crater margin. These lesions tend not to project outside the lumen. Sometimes gastric malignancy takes an infiltrative form and is referred to as 'linitis plastica' (Fig. 59). The normal mucosal pattern is destroyed and a narrow 'leather bottle' appearance is produced.

CT and ultrasound

Both CT and ultrasound can be used to assess the resectability of gastric cancer. Both techniques will evaluate the spread of the lesion outside the stomach, the presence of enlarged lymph nodes draining this area, and the presence of metastatic disease in the liver.

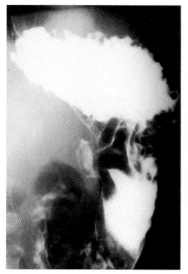

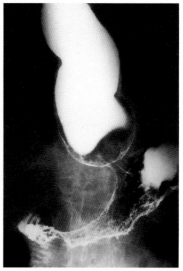

Fig. 58 Barium study showing lesser curve gastric ulcer.

Fig. 59 Linitis plastica.

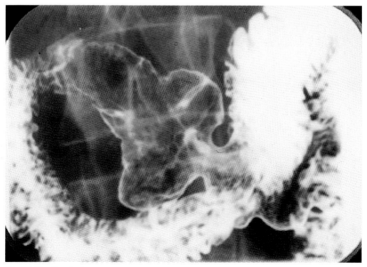

Fig. 60 Duodenal ulcer.

The small bowel

The small bowel may be demonstrated by following the barium column through from the stomach to the colon — the *barium follow-through* examination (Fig. 61). The transit time to the colon is in the region of 2–6 hours. The small bowel enema technique uses duodenal intubation to introduce barium and methyl cellulose, giving excellent mucosal detail.

Crohn's disease is the most common condition to affect the small bowel in the western world. In this condition, ulceration, strictures and mucosal disruption may be seen. The terminal ileum is frequently involved (Fig. 62). Abscess formation can occur. This may produce a mass effect and/or obstruction.

Meckel's diverticulum. This is the result of incomplete obliteration of the vitello-intestinal duct. It is present in up to 3% of the population and is usually located in the terminal ileum (Fig. 63). 60% of them contain gastric mucosa which may ulcerate and bleed. Some of these lesions may be demonstrated on barium studies. If the barium study is inconclusive, a ^{99m}Tc-pertechnetate scan may be useful, as this isotope when injected intravenously accumulates in gastric mucosa.

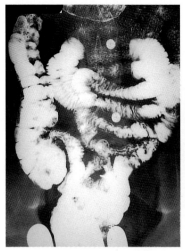

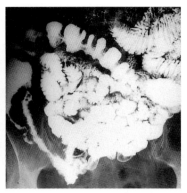

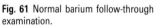

Fig. 61 Normal barium follow-through examination.

Fig. 62 Crohn's disease with ileal stricture.

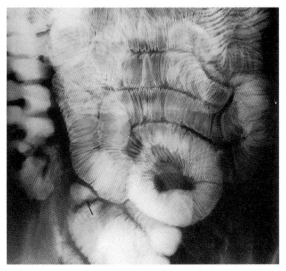

Fig. 63 Meckel's diverticulum in the distal ileum.

Colon and rectum

Contrast studies

The *double-contrast barium enema* involves the introduction of barium and air per rectum until the entire colon has been coated and distended. The best results are achieved when good preparation of the bowel has been obtained using a combination of a purgative and dietary restriction. Multiple films are obtained with the patient in different positions in order to obtain a clear view of the entire colon.

Colon cancer is the second commonest cancer. It arises in an adenoma which appears as a sessile or pedunculated filling defect in the barium study (Fig. 64). These lesions tend to occur most commonly in the rectosigmoid part of the colon. The larger the lesion, the greater the chance of malignancy within it. An established carcinoma appears as a filling defect or as an annular stricture with the so-called 'apple-core' configuration (Fig. 65).

Diverticular disease is a very common condition in the western world (Fig. 66). It may be complicated by abscess formation, fistulous communication to adjacent structures, bleeding or obstruction.

Colitis has many causes. During an acute episode, there may be considerable dilatation of the colon (Fig. 67) or perforation. Where the colitis is longstanding, the colon may be narrowed and tubular in appearance. There may be stricture formation. Shortening may be seen.

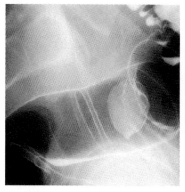

Fig. 64 Rectal polyp.

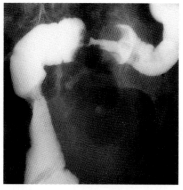

Fig. 65 Carcinoma of the rectosigmoid colon.

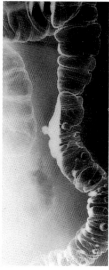

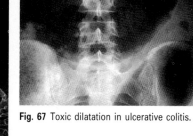

Fig. 67 Toxic dilatation in ulcerative colitis.

Fig. 66 Diverticular disease of the left side of the colon.

Investigation of gastrointestinal (GI) bleeding (Fig. 68)

Peptic ulceration, varices and erosions constitute the major sources of gastrointestinal bleeding in the upper GI tract, and diverticular disease, angiodysplasia and tumours in the lower GI tract.

Endoscopy and barium studies

The majority of patients who present with gastrointestinal bleeding will settle spontaneously with conservative measures. Endoscopic or barium studies can then be performed to establish the cause.

Angiography

In a small percentage of patients who present with acute severe bleeding and who do not respond to conservative measures, angiography may be used to localise the bleeding point. Both the superior and inferior mesenteric arteries are selected, and an examination of the coeliac axis and its branches is also included. Active bleeding is identified by the demonstration of extravasation of contrast at the bleeding site. Bleeding must be fairly brisk, around 0.5 ml per minute, for extravasation to be demonstrated.

Nuclear medicine

In those patients in whom conventional studies have not revealed a bleeding source, and where the bleeding is not brisk enough to be demonstrated by angiographic means or is intermittent, isotope studies may help. Either radioactive sulphur colloid or ^{99m}Tc-labelled red blood cells may be used. With the colloid, the isotope is removed from the circulation by the liver and spleen. If bleeding is occurring, this will be localised by a collection of the isotope at that site. The background activity will be low.

Alternatively, tracer-labelled red cells may show a leak of this isotope at the bleeding site.

^{99m}Tc-pertechnetate may be helpful where a Meckel's diverticulum is suspected (p. 43).

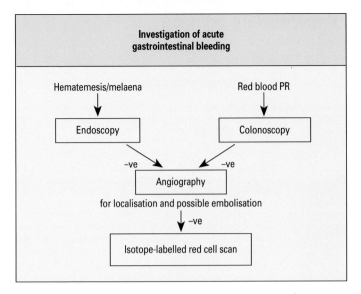

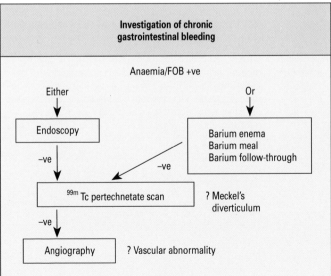

Fig. 68 Algorithm for investigation of GI bleeding.

5 / Hepatobiliary imaging

Gallstones in the gallbladder

Conventional radiology

Plain films are of limited value in the investigation of gallstone disease, only 15% of stones being radio-opaque (Figs 69, 70).

Ultrasound

Ultrasound is 90% accurate in the diagnosis of gallstones within the gallbladder. Typically they reflect the sound waves and produce a characteristic shadow posteriorly (Fig. 71). They will move about within the gallbladder.

Contrast studies

The oral cholecystogram is infrequently used, but may be of value when ultrasound is equivocal. This test involves the ingestion of an oral contrast agent which is absorbed through the gut, excreted into the bile and concentrated in the gallbladder. Failure to opacify the gallbladder will occur if there is malabsorption of the agent or poor liver function. Stones and polyps will show as negative defects in the opacified bile (Fig. 72).

Interventional radiology

Cholecystectomy by conventional or by laparoscopic means, is the primary mode of management of gallstones. Percutaneous cholecystostomy can be used for high risk patients with acute cholecystitis or empyema. Rarely, stones may be removed percutaneously using baskets and other mechanical devices.

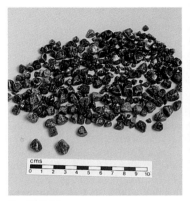

Fig. 69 Gallstones.

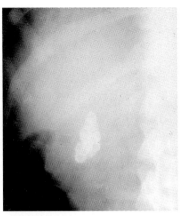

Fig. 70 Calcified stones seen on plain X-ray.

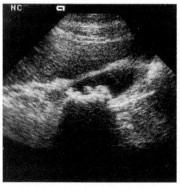

Fig. 71 Ultrasound showing typical echo from gallstones.

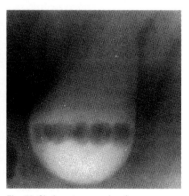

Fig. 72 Cholecystogram showing up non-opaque stones.

Gallstones in the duct system

Ultrasound

Duct stones may present with biliary colic or obstructive jaundice. The duct system is usually dilated. Ultrasound is the initial investigation of choice, being highly accurate in the evaluation of the intrahepatic and proximal extrahepatic duct system (Fig. 73).

Contrast studies

The definitive method of outlining the duct system is by introducing contrast material into it. This is done by *endoscopic retrograde cholangiopancreatography* (ERCP) (Fig. 74). In this procedure, an endoscope is passed through the oesophagus and stomach into the duodenum. The papilla is identified on the medial wall of the descending duodenum. A fine cannula is passed in and contrast introduced. This technique allows delineation of both the pancreatic duct and the biliary duct system.

Where the endoscopic approach to the bile ducts is not possible, a fine needle can be passed into the liver from the right mid-axillary position, between the ribs, using fluoroscopic guidance. Contrast is injected as the needle is slowly withdrawn until the biliary system is outlined; this is *percutaneous transhepatic cholangiography* (PTC; Fig. 75).

Interventional radiology

Stones in the duct system are generally managed by sphincterotomy and stone extraction. With very large stones, surgical removal may be required. In a few patients in whom surgery is considered to be too risky, *extracorporeal shock wave lithotripsy* may be useful. Ultrasound is used to localise the stones and shock-waves are directed to them. This may help to reduce the size of the stones which may then pass spontaneously or be rendered manageable by further sphincterotomy and basket extraction.

Stones retained in the duct system following cholecystectomy are also managed endoscopically. A T-tube is generally in place. Where endoscopic removal fails, the stones may be removed through the T-tube tract by passing a basket down the tract and into the duct system.

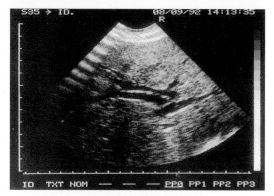

Fig. 73 Ultrasound showing dilated bile ducts.

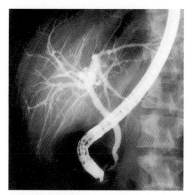

Fig. 74 Normal ERCP.

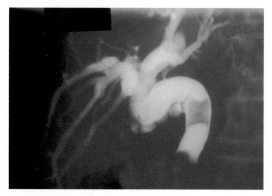

Fig. 75 PTC showing duct stones.

Benign biliary strictures

Aetiology

Benign strictures may be due to:
• congenital atresia
• trauma — mainly during gallbladder surgery
• post-inflammatory: secondary to gallstones, pancreatitis, duodenal ulcer, parasitic infection, recurrent cholangitis
• sclerosing cholangitis
• papillary stenosis.

Nuclear medicine

The secretion of the isotope ^{99m}Tc-labelled hepatoiminodiacetic acid (^{99m}Tc-HIDA) or disofenin is similar to that of bile. These isotopes can be useful when a biliary stricture is suspected, particularly where there has been a previous surgical procedure such as bilio-enteric anastomosis (Fig. 76).

Contrast studies

The ERCP is the definitive means of displaying the number and distribution of strictures. In sclerosing cholangitis (Fig. 77) the intrahepatic and extrahepatic ducts may be involved. Benign strictures have a smooth tapering appearance.

Interventional radiology

A papillary stenosis may be managed by endoscopic sphincterotomy. In sclerosing cholangitis, a focal dominant stricture may be dealt with by balloon dilatation or stenting.
   Where endoscopic management is not possible, a percutaneous approach may be used to provide access for dilatation or stenting. However, the majority of benign biliary strictures are best dealt with by surgical means.

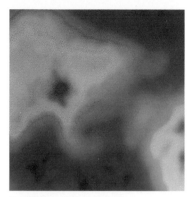

Fig. 76 Normal isotope scan.

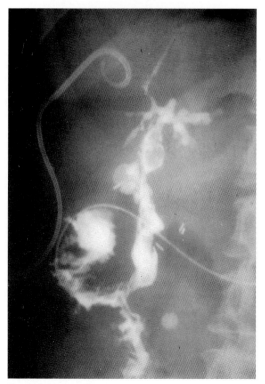

Fig. 77 Sclerosing cholangitis.

Malignant biliary strictures

Malignant obstruction of the distal bile duct may be due to an ampullary or pancreatic tumour (Fig. 78). With mid and high common bile duct strictures, gallbladder carcinoma, cholangiocarcinoma (Fig. 79) or involvement of the duct system by malignant nodes should be considered.

Ultrasound Ultrasound may show a mass lesion with proximal dilatation of the duct system, and biopsy can be performed under ultrasound guidance.

CT CT scanning offers a more detailed study of intra- and extrahepatic structures and will aid in the assessment of resectability.

Contrast studies ERCP portrays the pancreatic ducts in addition to the biliary system. The papilla can be inspected and biopsied if necessary. A focal stricture may be evident in both pancreatic and biliary duct systems when there is a pancreatic carcinoma affecting the head of the gland.

Interventional radiology Decompression of an obstructed biliary system can be achieved endoscopically by introducing a guidewire into the system and then advancing a stent into it. The tubes may be open wire-mesh stents (Fig. 80) similar to those used in the arterial system, or multi-holed plastic tubes (Fig. 81). The plastic tubes tend to become blocked by food debris. They have a patency of around 3 months at which time they can be exchanged endoscopically. The wire-mesh stents are permanent. They are much wider and are blocked by tumour ingrowth or overgrowth rather than by food. They have a longer patency, of around 10 months, and are therefore preferable.

Where the endoscopic approach to the bile ducts is unsuccessful, a percutaneous technique can be used. Using the same method as for PTC and using fluoroscopic guidance, a needle is introduced into the biliary system. A guidewire is advanced through the needle to the duodenum. The liver tract is dilated and a stent introduced over the guidewire to the desired position.

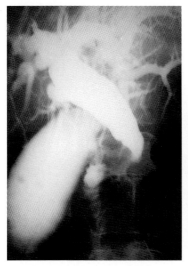

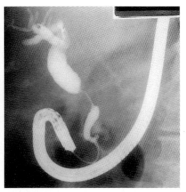

Fig. 78 Stricture due to pancreatic carcinoma.

Fig. 79 Cholangiocarcinoma.

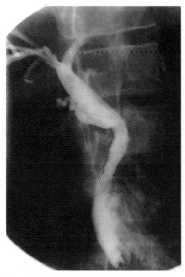

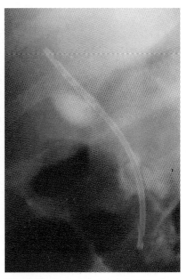

Fig. 80 Metal stent inserted. Same patient as Figure 78.

Fig. 81 Plastic stent inserted. Same patient as Figure 79.

Benign liver tumours

Benign liver tumours may not produce any symptoms but may be detected incidentally during radiological examination or at surgery. Some may grow so large that they produce a mass effect, while a few may cause acute symptoms due to necrosis or haemorrhage. They include haemangiomas, cysts and adenomas.

Ultrasound On ultrasound, haemangiomas are usually subcapsular in position and bright or hyperechoic (Fig. 82). Cysts, on the other hand, have a clear-cut margin, and have no internal solid components and are therefore anechoic. Adenomas are also well-defined lesions. They have a variable echo pattern.

CT On CT scanning, haemangiomas are of low attenuation, appearing as black holes against the normal liver parenchyma. However, when intravenous contrast is administered, they have a characteristic appearance. The margin enhances, or lights up, as contrast collects in the periphery of the lesion. Contrast permeates to the centre of the lesion and is retained in it well after it has passed through the rest of the liver. This delayed contrast retention is a characteristic feature of these lesions.

Cysts appear as thin-walled non-enhancing fluid dense structures (Fig. 83).

Adenomas are often encapsulated. They tend to enhance with intravenous contrast. They may be indistinguishable from hepatocellular carcinoma.

MRI MRI may be helpful in characterising some liver tumours. Haemangiomas, for example, have a characteristic bright appearance, sometimes likened to a 'light bulb' (Fig. 84).

Angiography Where the other less invasive procedures have failed to characterise a lesion, angiography may be helpful. Haemangiomas have a typical angiographic appearance with pooling of contrast in the large vascular channels.

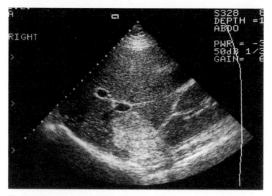

Fig. 82 Ultrasound showing haemangioma.

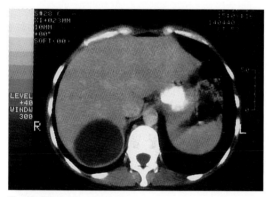

Fig. 83 CT showing simple liver cyst.

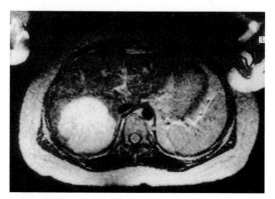

Fig. 84 MRI showing haemangioma.

Malignant liver tumours

Primary hepatocellular carcinoma generally occurs against a background of chronic liver disease or hepatitis B.

Ultrasound   On ultrasound the lesion may be solitary, multiple or diffusely infiltrating. It may be hyperechoic (bright) or hypoechoic (dark). The tumour tends to grow along the portal vein and it may be possible to demonstrate tumour involvement of this vessel on ultrasound.

CT   On CT the lesion may not be clearly seen without intravenous contrast administration. It may be encapsulated. Associated features of cirrhosis, with irregularity of the liver outline and portal hypertension with splenomegaly and enlarged collateral venous channels may be evident.

Angiography   Hepatocellular carcinoma is generally very vascular (Fig. 85). Arterio-venous shunting may be present. Tumour in the portal veins may be evident.

MRI   The role of MRI is yet to be established (Fig. 86).

Metastases

These are the most common malignant liver tumours. On ultrasound they may be single or multiple and have a variable appearance (Fig. 87).

Liver resection may be possible depending on the site and size of the lesions. Ultrasound and CT (Fig. 88) are useful in staging the disease.

Interventional radiology   Resection offers the best prognosis. Where surgery is not possible, chemotherapy may be considered. This may be delivered directly into the hepatic artery supplying the tumour, and combined with an agent which will occlude the artery. This is accomplished in the same manner as in angiography; it is called transarterial chemoembolisation. Small tumours may be treated by percutaneous injection of alcohol carried out under ultrasound guidance.

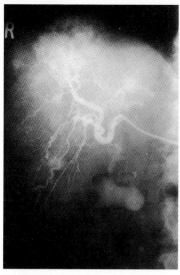

Fig. 85 Angiogram showing multifocal hepatoma.

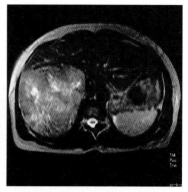

Fig. 86 MRI showing hepatoma.

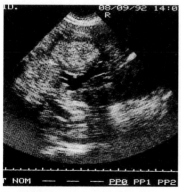

Fig. 87 Ultrasound showing liver metastases.

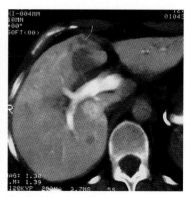

Fig. 88 CT showing liver metastases.

The investigation of obstructive jaundice (Fig. 89)

Ultrasound   The initial examination of the patient with obstructive jaundice is an ultrasound study of the upper abdomen. This will demonstrate whether or not the biliary duct system is dilated. Where there is no dilatation, a liver biopsy may provide the diagnosis. However, it should be borne in mind that a small stone may be present in the biliary system without duct dilatation. If liver biopsy is unhelpful, a cholangiogram should be obtained, usually by ERCP, to ensure that there is no stone in the system.

Contrast studies   Where there is biliary dilatation, cholangiography is indicated. In most instances this will be carried out by ERCP or where that is not feasible, by PTC. Cholangiography will localise and characterise the obstruction.

Interventional therapy   Mention has already been made of the options for endoscopic or percutaneous management of stones and tumours obstructing the biliary system (pp. 51, 53, 55).

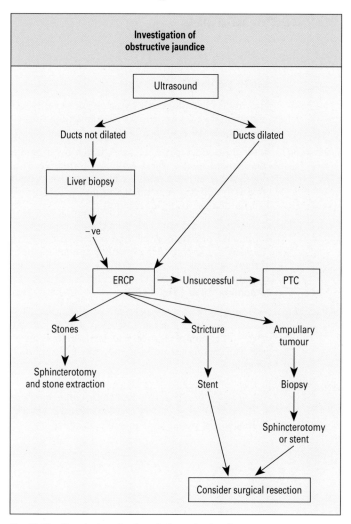

Fig. 89 Algorithm for investigation of obstructive jaundice.

6 / Pancreatic imaging

Acute pancreatitis

The role of radiology is in staging the severity of the inflammatory process and in the detection and management of complications.

Ultrasound

Both ultrasound and CT may show a focal or diffuse enlargement of the gland, with the formation of an ill-defined indurated mass (a phlegmon) or a fluid collection. Biliary duct dilatation and gallstones will also be defined using ultrasound.

CT

CT is the investigation of choice and will show the extent and distribution of fluid collections (Fig. 90). Necrosis is indicated by nonenhancement of the gland during an intravenous contrast injection. Haemorrhage appears hyperdense on CT, an abscess as a gas-containing mass (Fig. 91).

Angiography

Angiography will show vascular complications. In 10% of cases, pseudoaneurysms develop due to extension of the inflammatory process to involve adjacent arteries. Venous thrombosis may affect the portal system.

Interventional radiology

Stones in the biliary system can be removed endoscopically. Abscesses and fluid collections can be drained. Percutaneous cyst-gastrostomy allows drainage of a pseudocyst into the stomach.

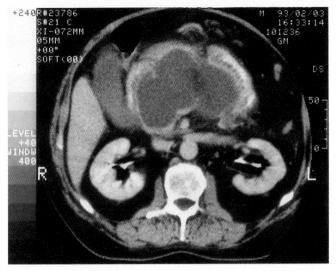

Fig. 90 CT showing fluid collection around the pancreas.

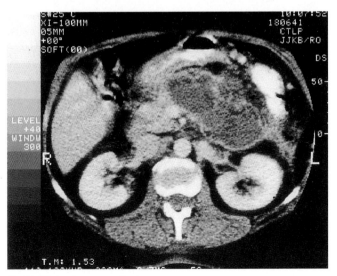

Fig. 91 CT showing pancreatic abscess.

Chronic pancreatitis

A continuation of pancreatic inflammation leads
to irreversible damage. Alcohol and stones are the
usual contributing factors. Radiological investigations
are aimed at evaluating the severity of the disease and
the associated complications, and aiding in pre-
operative assessment.

Conventional radiology
Calcification is seen in the region of the pancreas on
the supine abdominal film (Fig. 92).

Ultrasound and CT
Both ultrasound and CT may show a change in gland
size, either focal or diffuse. Eventually, atrophy of the
gland will occur. On CT, calcification (Fig. 93) along
with pancreatic or biliary duct dilatation may be
evident.

ERCP
The pancreatic duct typically shows areas of dilatation
and stenosis (Fig. 94). Concretions may be seen
within the duct system. An associated stricture of the
common bile duct is seen in 10%.

Interventional radiology
Patients with biliary calculi should have a
sphincterotomy. Occasionally, pancreatic drainage may
be helped by the insertion of a stent across a duct
stricture.

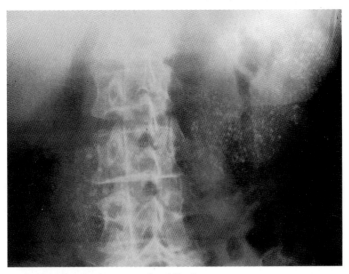

Fig. 92 Plain film showing pancreatic calcification.

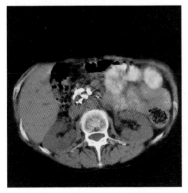

Fig. 93 CT showing atrophic calcified pancreas.

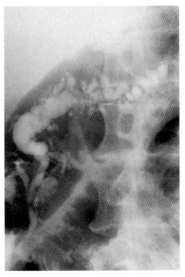

Fig. 94 ERCP showing pancreatic duct changes of chronic pancreatitis.

Benign pancreatic tumours

Ultrasound and CT

Tumours greater than 2 cm in diameter are detected by *ultrasound* or *CT scanning*. However, the detection of smaller lesions may require sophisticated and invasive investigations, including *angiography* and *transhepatic portal venous sampling*. In this latter technique, a needle is inserted into the liver in the same manner as for PTC (p. 51). Contrast is injected as the needle is slowly withdrawn. When the contrast outlines portal branches, a guidewire and catheter are advanced into the portal system. Blood samples can be obtained from the numerous branches around the pancreas. Hormone assay of these samples can help to localise an endocrine lesion.

Cystic lesions. Most pancreatic cystic lesions are the result of inflammation or trauma. Multicystic or complex lesions should raise the suspicion of a tumour rather than a simple cyst.

Malignant pancreatic tumours

Ultrasound and CT

Adenocarcinoma is the commonest malignant tumour of the pancreas, and 60% occur in the head of the gland. A focal mass may be seen on *ultrasound* or *CT* (Fig. 95). Dilatation of the pancreatic duct upstream from the tumour may be seen. The biliary system is also frequently dilated when the lesion is in the head of the pancreas. *ERCP* usually shows a focal occlusion of the pancreatic duct (Fig. 96). A corresponding stricture or occlusion of the common bile duct is frequently seen — the double duct sign.

Invasion of major vascular structures is the main factor precluding curative resection. Involvement of these structures can be detected by CT.

Interventional radiology

Percutaneous biopsy under ultrasound or CT guidance may be used to obtain histological proof of cancer. Biliary stenting by either endoscopic or percutaneous means is frequently used to relieve jaundice and itch prior to surgery, or as a definitive measure where surgery is not contemplated.

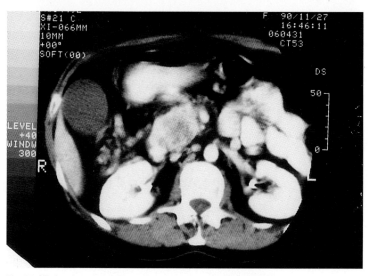

Fig. 95 CT showing pancreatic carcinoma in the head of the gland.

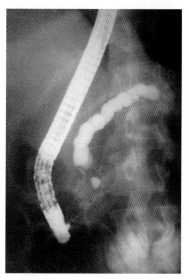

Fig. 96 ERCP showing stenosis of the pancreatic duct due to carcinoma.

7 / Urological imaging

Ultrasound Ultrasound provides a safe and accurate means of assessing the urinary system. Obstruction of the collecting system can be accurately diagnosed. The level of obstruction and its cause may not be clearly shown. However, ultrasound should be the initial modality employed in the evaluation of a suspected urinary problem.

Contrast studies The *intravenous urogram* (IVU) provides an anatomical display of the urinary system. Plain films of the abdomen, to include kidneys, ureters and bladder, are obtained initially. These allow the detection of calcification. Following an intravenous injection of contrast medium, further views are obtained, the contrast excretion delineating the urinary tract.

Infection

Acute pyelonephritis is frequently the result of ascending infection. Vesico-ureteric reflux and obstruction both predispose to infection. The kidney may be normal or enlarged. Any obstruction, its level and aetiology will be demonstrated on the IVU.
Renal abscess (Fig. 97). This may occur if an infection is inadequately treated. Diabetics and drug abusers are more prone to abscess formation. On ultrasound or on the IVU, a mass is identified. It may displace the collecting system, and is usually ill-defined and solid. On the control IVU films, a mottled appearance is characteristic.
Chronic pyelonephritis. The kidneys gradually become smaller and scarred (Fig. 98). The calyces may be distorted.
Tuberculosis. Distorted calyces associated with calcification raises the possibility of tuberculosis. Associated changes seen on urography and ultrasound include ureteric strictures and hydronephrosis.

Interventional radiology Under ultrasound or fluoroscopic guidance, abscess drainage can be performed. An obstructed or infected collecting system can be decompressed and drained.

69

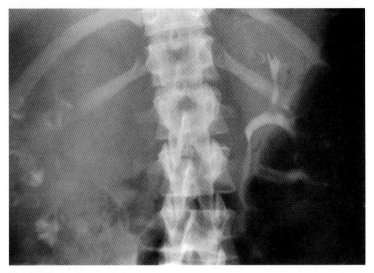

Fig. 97 IVU showing renal abscess.

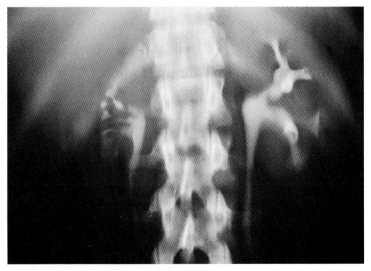

Fig. 98 IVU showing renal scarring.

Stones

Conventional radiology

The majority of renal stones are radio-opaque, as they contain calcium oxalate and phosphate. They are thus readily visible on the plain films (Fig. 99).

Contrast studies

An IVU will show the relationship of the stones to the system, and any secondary obstructive changes (Fig. 100). An acute ureteric obstruction is usually due to a stone. The less common nonopaque stones are seen as filling defects in the contrast study.

Bladder stones tend to occur when there is obstruction to the bladder outflow, e.g. when there is enlargement of the prostate or perhaps a urethral stricture. These may grow to considerable size.

Ultrasound will show dilatation of the collecting system proximal to an obstructing stone, but it is not as good as the IVU in demonstrating the level of obstruction. On the obstructed side, in addition to the dilated urinary system above the stone, the renal parenchyma may appear particularly dense on the IVU and where the obstruction is acute, extravasation of contrast may be observed.

Interventional radiology

Most small stones generally pass spontaneously. Larger stones have to be removed. This can be done by the urologist passing an endoscope called a cystoscope into the bladder per urethram, and passing a basket device up the ureter to retrieve the stone. When this cannot be performed, the stone may be retrieved by basket extraction using a percutaneous approach to the collecting system. A needle is introduced percutaneously into the system using fluoroscopic or ultrasound guidance. A guidewire is then advanced, and the tract to the kidney dilated. A large-bore tube is passed over the guidewire into the system and a basket device used to retrieve the stone.

Where the stone is very large, surgery may be required. Extracorporeal shock-wave lithotripsy may be used to reduce the size of the stone. Alternatively, an electrohydraulic lithotriptor may be introduced percutaneously and placed in contact with the stone to fragment it (Fig. 101).

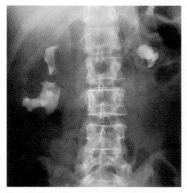

Fig. 99 Plain film showing calcified stones.

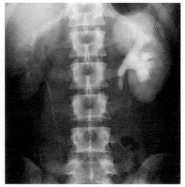

Fig. 100 IVU showing calculous obstruction of left ureter.

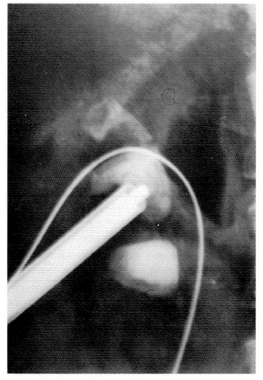

Fig. 101 Electrohydraulic lithotriptor used to fragment stones.

Benign tumours

Ultrasound During ultrasound examination, small benign renal tumours, such as adenomas, may be observed incidentally. These appear as well-defined, solid focal masses. Renal cysts are also found incidentally. They also have a sharp interface with normal renal tissue but are fluid-filled with no internal echo pattern.

IVU On the IVU, benign tumours appear as well-defined masses. Ultrasound is required to establish whether these lesions are cystic or solid.

Malignant tumours

Renal tumours

Ultrasound Adenocarcinoma is the commonest renal tumour, accounting for 90% of cases. On ultrasound these lesions are not well-defined. They are solid. The tumour may extend along the renal vein to the inferior vena cava and this feature may be detected by ultrasound.

Contrast study On the IVU a mass is seen distorting or displacing the collecting system. There is usually some renal function.

CT On CT a solid mass is evident (Fig. 102). There is no sharp interface with normal renal tissue. CT is useful in assessing spread of the lesion outside the renal capsule and in identifying enlarged lymph nodes.

Bladder tumours

Bladder tumours may also be identified on ultrasound. On the IVU a filling defect may be seen (Fig. 103). Lesions smaller than 5 mm cannot be seen however. CT is the optimal way of staging bladder tumours. It will demonstrate extravesical spread of the lesion and nodal enlargement.

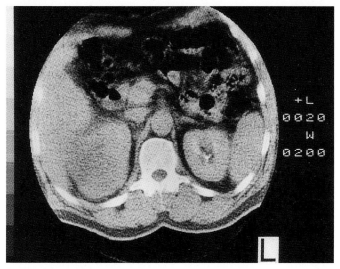

Fig. 102 CT showing renal carcinoma.

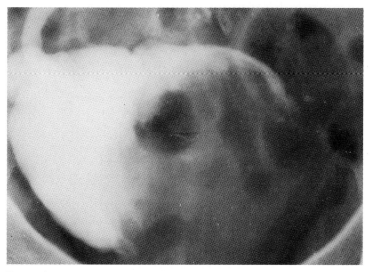

Fig. 103 Cystogram showing large bladder carcinoma.

Renovascular hypertension

In 4–5% hypertensive patients there is a renovascular cause. This is usually renal artery stenosis (RAS) resulting from atheroma, or in young women it may be due to fibromuscular hyperplasia.

Contrast studies Signs on the IVU suggesting renal ischaemia include a dense pyelogram and a small kidney, but the findings are not specific.

Nuclear medicine Renography, using intravenous ^{99m}Tc-DTPA (dimethyl tri-ethyl penta acetate), has been used in the evaluation of hypertensive patients. The agent collects in the nephrons, producing a rise in activity in the first few minutes reflecting renal perfusion. There is a peak activity normally within 3–5 minutes, and over the ensuing 20 minutes a gradual fall. In RAS the curve is flatter and lower than normal. With bilateral stenosis, or where the stenosis affects a branch artery, the results are confusing.

Angiography An aortogram is the definitive means of demonstrating the vascular supply to the kidneys.

Interventional radiology Where RAS is demonstrated angiographically (Fig. 104), angioplasty (Figs 105, 106) or stenting may be useful.

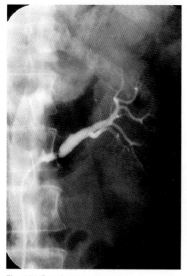

Fig. 104 Renal artery stenosis.

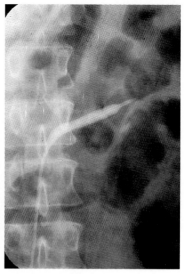

Fig. 105 Angioplasty balloon in place.

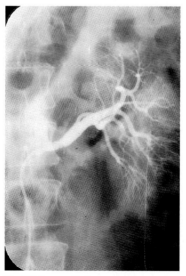

Fig. 106 Post-angioplasty result.

Trauma

Conventional radiology
Renal trauma is usually related to road traffic accidents, to a penetrating injury such as stabbing or it may follow renal biopsy. Where there are fractures of the lower ribs or the transverse processes of vertebrae in the thoraco-lumbar area, a renal injury should be suspected.

Contrast studies
It is essential to inject a high dose (at least 100 ml) of contrast. Films are obtained immediately in order to obtain an optimal view of the renal outlines. The injured kidney may be swollen, ill defined or may function poorly. If the renal vascular pedicle has been completely avulsed, no function will be seen. Where the kidney is fractured, frank extravasation of contrast may be seen (Fig. 107).

Pelvic fractures (Fig. 108) may be associated with bladder or urethral injuries. Where an injury of this nature is suspected, contrast is introduced into the bladder by urethral or suprapubic catheter (cystography); there will be extravasation of contrast if a rupture is present (Fig. 109). In the presence of pelvic fractures, the bladder may be compressed by urine and blood, giving it a 'tear-drop' configuration on the cystogram.

CT
Contrast-enhanced CT scanning will show renal injuries. It is particularly good in the demonstration of subcapsular haematomas. Other soft tissue injuries and undetected skeletal injuries may also be evident.

Angiography
Where avulsion of the renal vascular pedicle is suspected, angiography is indicated. This will show an occlusion of the artery to the injured kidney.

Interventional radiology
Pelvic fractures are associated with considerable blood loss. When the patient is unstable with continuing blood loss, angiography may be helpful in localising a bleeding artery. Bleeding may be arrested by introducing embolic material into the bleeding vessel in order to occlude it, a procedure called embolisation.

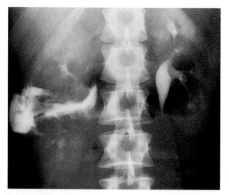

Fig. 107 IVU with renal disruption.

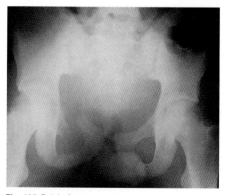

Fig. 108 Pelvic fracture — suspect bladder injury.

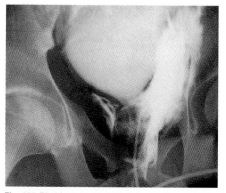

Fig. 109 Bladder rupture with extravasation of contrast.

8 / Musculoskeletal imaging

Conventional radiology

Plain films remain the mainstay of musculoskeletal diagnosis. The high atomic number and density of calcium in the bone mineral accounts for the visibility of bone on plain radiographs.

Fractures give rise to breaks in the continuity of the cortex (Fig. 110); there may be angulation and displacement. When the diagnosis is difficult, an isotope scan will show increased uptake at the fracture site (see below). Bone resorption will result in the fracture line becoming more obvious on a repeat film after two weeks.

Nuclear medicine

Isotope bone scanning using ^{99m}Tc-phosphate and diphosphonate identifies areas of active bone metabolism. Thus, osteomyelitis, fractures and most malignant bone tumours appear 'hot', whereas benign inactive lesions are 'cold'. The scan appearance is nonspecific, and correlation with radiographs is essential.

MRI

MRI is the imaging modality of choice in many musculoskeletal applications, particularly in knee-cartilage tears (Fig. 111), lumbar disc disease (Fig. 112) and the staging of malignant tumours.

CT

CT scanning has a role in complex trauma, providing information regarding the soft tissues adjacent to the fractures and detecting previously undiagnosed skeletal injuries. It is also used in the evaluation of lumbar disc disease where MRI is not available.

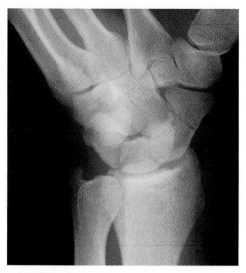

Fig. 110 Fractured scaphoid.

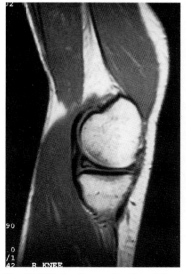

Fig. 111 MRI showing meniscal knee injury.

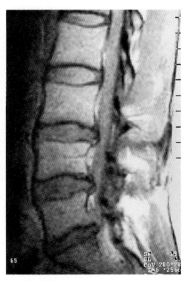

Fig. 112 MRI showing lumbar disc disease.

Infection

Acute osteomyelitis

Conventional radiology

Acute osteomyelitis is a blood-borne infection which usually affects the metaphysis of long bones in childhood. No abnormality may be detectable on plain radiographs. The initial changes are in the soft tissues, with blurring of tissue planes due to oedema, followed by periosteal new bone formation.

Nuclear medicine

The isotope bone scan is positive from the outset (Fig. 113), due to hyperaemia and increased osteoblast activity.

Chronic osteomyelitis

Chronic osteomyelitis is characterised by necrotic, infected bone (sequestrum) surrounded by a shell of new bone (involucrum) (Fig. 114).

Septic arthritis

Conventional radiology

Septic arthritis gives rise to joint effusion with widening of the joint space (Fig. 115). Progressive destruction of the articular surface occurs, which, if untreated, heals by joint fusion.

Tuberculosis

Conventional radiology

Tuberculosis of the spine causes loss of disc height with progressive destruction of the adjacent vertebral bodies, typically resulting in marked angulation. Associated paraspinal abscesses may calcify (Fig. 116).

Tuberculosis may also affect the limb joints and, in childhood, the chronic hyperaemia leads to early fusion of the growth plate, resulting in limb shortening.

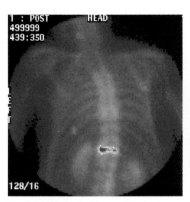

Fig. 113 'Hot spot' on isotope bone scan.

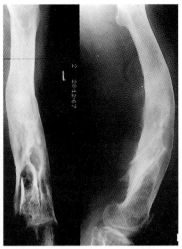

Fig. 114 Chronic osteomyelitis of the femur.

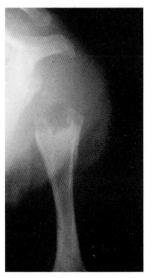

Fig. 115 Septic arthritis of the left shoulder in a child.

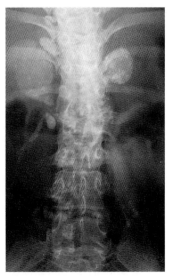

Fig. 116 Chronic TB of the spine.

Benign tumours

Conventional radiology

Benign bone tumours are generally well defined (Figs 117, 118). The bone may be expanded. Expansion is gross in an aneurysmal bone cyst.

Nuclear medicine

A bone lesion which is 'cold' on isotope scan is generally benign, but the converse is not true. Some benign tumours, e.g. osteoid osteoma, are 'hot', as are benign lesions due to trauma and infection.

Malignant tumours (primary)

Primary malignant bone tumours usually affect the long bones in children and young adults. The hallmarks include elevation of the periosteum, bone destruction, a soft tissue mass, and increased uptake on the isotope bone scan.

MRI is the most sensitive imaging modality.

Osteogenic sarcoma arises in the metaphyseal region. It is of variable density due to tumour bone formation. Periosteal reaction may take the form of 'Codman's triangles' at the site of elevation of the periosteum from the cortex, or of radiating spicules of bone (Fig. 119).

Ewing's sarcoma arises in the diaphysis. It elevates the periosteum, resulting in laminar periosteal new bone and Codman's triangles.

Malignant tumours (secondary)

Secondary deposits may be sclerotic (high density) or lytic (low density; Fig. 120). The isotope bone scan typically shows multiple 'hot' spots.

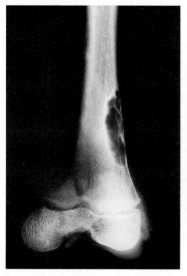

Fig. 117 Benign fibrous cortical defect.

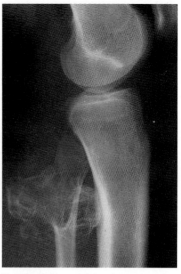

Fig. 118 Benign osteochondroma.

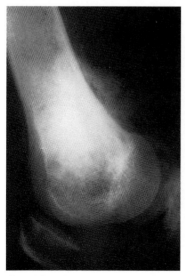

Fig. 119 Primary osteosarcoma.

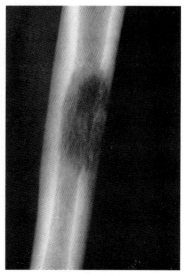

Fig. 120 Lytic metastatic deposit in femur.

Metabolic bone disease

Conventional radiology

Osteomalacia. This results from deficiency of the active form of vitamin D, due to poor diet, malabsorption, renal or liver disease. There is an excess of nonossified bone matrix, with reduced density and weakening of bones resulting in deformity. Partial cortical fractures (Looser's zones) occur. In childhood, the bone changes are called rickets (Fig. 121). Bone matrix at the growth plate fails to ossify, resulting in a wide radiolucent band. The weakened metaphysis is splayed and cupped, and the diaphysis is bowed.

Hyperparathyroidism. Excess production of parathyroid hormone leads to mobilisation of calcium from the bones, manifest as subperiosteal bone resorption, resorption of the tufts of the phalanges, and lytic lesions ('brown tumours'). Hypercalcaemia leads to soft tissue calcification.

Bone disease in chronic renal failure results from abnormal vitamin D metabolism, hyperparathyroidism and impaired renal phosphate excretion. Calcium deposition adjacent to the vertebral end plates gives a 'rugger-jersey spine' (Fig. 122).

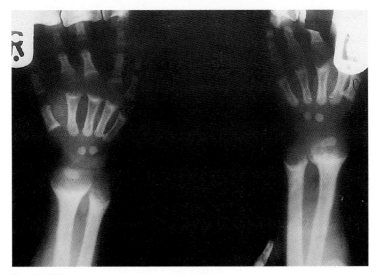

Fig. 121 Rickets.

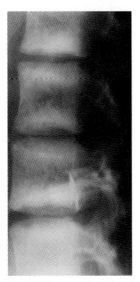

Fig. 122 Hyperparathyroidism: 'rugger jersey' spine.

Joints

Osteoarthritis commonly affects the weight-bearing joints. Loss of cartilage leads to reduction in the joint space. There is subarticular sclerosis. Beaks of bone occur at the joint margin (osteophytes) (Fig. 123).

Rheumatoid arthritis commonly affects the metacarpophalangeal joints, but any synovial joint may be involved. Inflammation produces swelling and hyperaemia, resulting in widening of the joint space and peri-articular osteopenia. Later, bone erosion occurs at the joint margin. Ligament laxity results in deformity, with ulnar deviation of the fingers (Fig. 124).

Ankylosing spondylitis is commonest in young males and presents with back pains and stiffness. The sacro-iliac joints and spine are mainly affected (Fig. 125). The sacro-iliac joints may initally appear hazy or ill-defined, and later become sclerotic. The end-result may be bony ankylosis. Ossification of the spinal ligaments results in 'bamboo spine'.

Neuropathic arthropathy results from absence of pain sensation and consequent repeated minor trauma with joint destruction and disruption.

Gout is due to urate crystal deposition in the synovium. The inflammation results in soft tissue swelling and, when chronic, well-defined bone erosions and soft tissue masses (tophi) (Fig. 126).

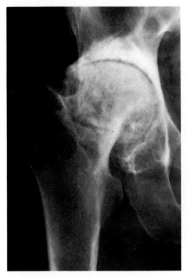

Fig. 123 Osteoarthritis of the hip.

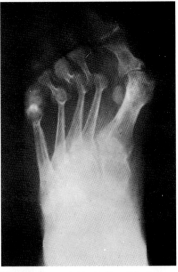

Fig. 124 Rheumatoid arthritis of the feet.

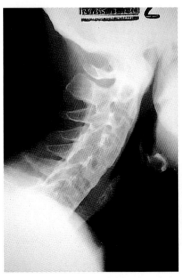

Fig. 125 Ankylosing spondylitis of cervical spine.

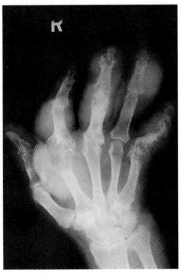

Fig. 126 Gouty arthropathy.

Miscellaneous

Paget's disease. This is a common disease of the elderly of unknown aetiology. It usually affects the axial skeleton and proximal limb bones. An initial zone of osteolysis in the active phase is followed by thickening of the cortex and a coarse trabecular pattern (Fig. 127). The bone is weakened, causing bowing. The affected bones show increased uptake in the isotope bone scan. Sarcoma occurs in 1%.

Fibrous dysplasia. This is a common finding in children and young adults (Fig. 128). Normal bone is replaced by a region of partially calcified fibrous tissue. Common sites include the proximal femora and ribs. There is expansion of the bone with weakening resulting, for example, in the 'shepherd's crook' deformity of the femoral neck.

Haemophilia. This is a hereditary disorder of the clotting system which is complicated by recurrent bleeding into large joints. The resulting hyperaemia in childhood causes overgrowth of the epiphysis, but also limb shortening due to premature fusion of the growth plate. There is synovial hypertrophy which causes loss of cartilage, joint erosions and premature degenerative changes (Fig. 129).

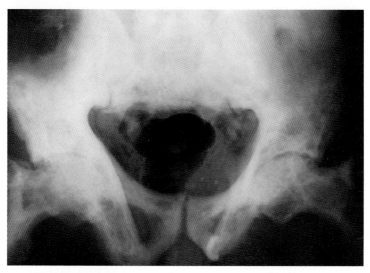

Fig. 127 Paget's disease of pelvis.

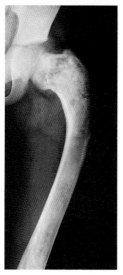

Fig. 128 Fibrous dysplasia of proximal femur.

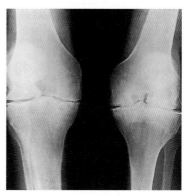

Fig. 129 Haemophilic joint disease.

9 / Neurological imaging

Cerebrovascular disease: ischaemia and haemorrhage

CT   A CT scan of the head is the initial means of investigating the patient who has sustained an acute cerebrovascular accident. This is done without the administration of intravenous contrast material. It will differentiate haemorrhage from infarct.

Cerebral infarction does not become apparent for up to 48 hours, at which stage a low-attenuation (dark) area is seen at the site of the infarct.
Cerebral haemorrhage. An acute cerebral haemorrhage is identified by the presence of a high-attenuation (white) area in the brain parenchyma (Fig. 130). If the haemorrhage is large, there may be a mass effect, with displacement of adjacent structures. Subarachnoid haemorrhage is identified by the presence of high attenuation blood in the subarachnoid space. The usual cause is rupture of an aneurysm (Fig. 132). Following subdural haemorrhage, blood forms a crescent over the convexity of the brain. An extradural haemorrhage is restricted by the firm attachment of the dura to the skull, typically producing a biconvex haematoma.

Doppler ultrasound   Transient ischaemic attacks may occur prior to the onset of a major cerebrovascular infarction. These events may result from stenosis or plaque formation at the carotid bifurcation. The extracranial carotid circulation can be studied using Doppler ultrasound.

Angiography   Conventional or digital angiography (Fig. 131) gives better anatomical detail of the intracranial and extracranial vascular structures than Doppler imaging. A catheter is introduced percutaneously into the femoral artery and advanced to the arch of the aorta. Views of the origins of the head and neck arteries can be obtained prior to selective catheterisation of the vessels of particular interest.

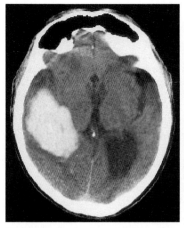

Fig. 130 CT showing intracerebral haemorrhage.

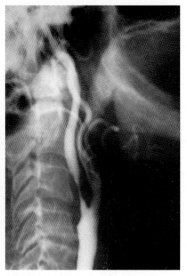

Fig. 131 Angiogram showing carotid stenosis.

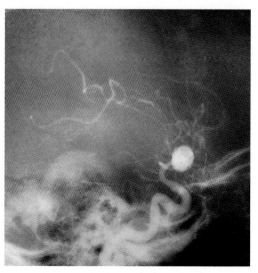

Fig. 132 Angiogram showing cerebral aneurysm.

CT   ***Cerebral abscesses***. These may be single or
multiple. Typically they appear on CT scanning as a
low-attenuation (dark) area against the normal brain
tissue. As with other intracerebral mass lesions, they
may displace adjacent and mid-line structures.
Following an intravenous contrast injection, they
exhibit peripheral ring enhancement (Fig. 133).
However, these appearances are not specific and
differentiation from a primary or secondary tumour is
usually made clinically.

MRI   ***Multiple sclerosis*** is characterised by multiple
plaques of demyelination in the central nervous
system. Occasionally, plaques may be demonstrated
on CT. However, MRI is much more sensitive in the
detection of plaques and is the imaging modality of
choice (Fig. 134).

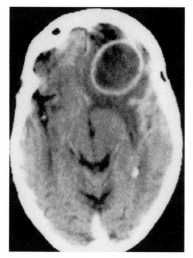

Fig. 133 CT showing a cerebral abscess.

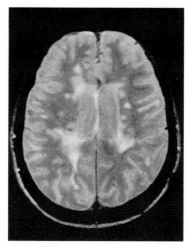

Fig. 134 MRI showing plaques of multiple sclerosis.

Intracranial tumours

Conventional radiology

Plain films are of little value in the initial investigation of intracranial mass lesions. Changes due to raised intracranial pressure, such as erosion of the bony cortex of the dorsum sellae or focal thickening of the bone due to an adjacent meningioma, may occasionally be seen.

CT and MRI

Both CT and MRI are useful in the evaluation of intracranial tumours. The brainstem and cerebellum are closely encased in the bone which impairs the image quality of CT. However, bone gives no signal on MRI so this is the modality of choice, particularly when examining the posterior fossa.

Primary gliomas. These have a broad spectrum of CT appearances. Calcification within the tumour suggests a slow-growing, benign type of lesion. Malignant lesions show irregular enhancement following intravenous contrast injection, and are surrounded by a dark area of oedema (Fig. 135).

MRI appearances also vary. Both tumour and oedema give rise to a high-intensity signal (white or bright) (Fig. 136). Calcification produces no signal and is hard to detect on MRI.

Meningiomas. These are benign tumours arising in relation to the meninges at characteristic sites, most commonly related to the sphenoid ridge, the falx and the convex surface of the brain. They are of high attenuation (bright or white) on CT but low signal intensity (dark) on MRI. *Angiography* shows them to be very vascular lesions (Fig. 137).

Cerebral metastases usually show intense enhancement and marked surrounding oedema on CT. They are often multiple.

Acoustic neuromas arise from the eighth cranial nerve. They may cause expansion of the internal auditory meatus, which is detectable on CT scanning (Fig. 138).

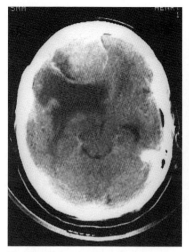

Fig. 135 CT showing cerebral tumour.

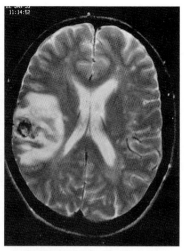

Fig. 136 MRI showing cerebral tumour.

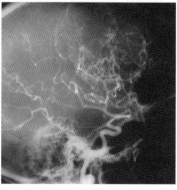

Fig. 137 Angiogram showing tumour circulation.

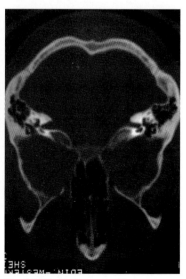

Fig. 138 CT showing acoustic neuroma.

Spine

Conventional radiology
Plain films of the lumbar spine are frequently undertaken for back pain and sciatica, but are rarely helpful. Degenerative changes are frequently present.

CT
Axial CT slices through the lumbar discs reveal disc prolapse as a bulge of high-attenuation disc material impinging on the spinal canal (Fig. 139).

Contrast studies
Myelography requires injection of contrast medium into the subarachnoid space around the spinal cord and cauda equina via lumbar puncture. A disc prolapse is shown as an anterior indentation of the thecal sac. A small lateral disc prolapse may only cause kinking or thickening of the affected nerve root or underfilling of the nerve root sleeve (Fig. 140). Myelography is frequently complicated by unpleasant headache, so CT or MRI is preferred.

MRI
MRI is the imaging modality of choice in disc disease (Fig. 141) and other spinal cord pathology.

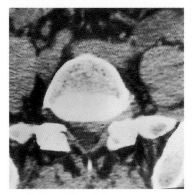

Fig. 139 CT of disc disease.

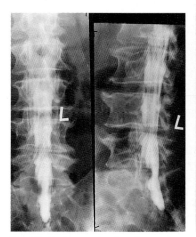

Fig. 140 Myelogram showing disc protrusion.

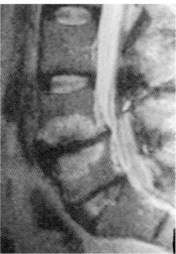

Fig. 141 MRI of disc disease.

10 / **Obstetric imaging**

Ultrasound Exposure of the gravid uterus to radiation should be avoided because of the risk of carcinogenesis and mental retardation in the fetus. Assessment of the fetus by ultrasound has become routine in antenatal care (Fig. 142). It is believed to be harmless. In early pregnancy, a full bladder is essential to provide a window into the pelvis.

Ultrasound can demonstrate the fetal heart beat at 6 weeks gestation. The number of fetuses and the location of the gestational sac (intra-uterine or ectopic) is readily assessed. Up to 12 weeks gestation, the age of the fetus can be accurately assessed by measurement of its crown–rump and femur length. From 12–28 weeks, biparietal diameter is used.

In placental insufficiency, the fetal head usually grows at the normal rate whereas the body is abnormally small. Placental abnormalities, such as placenta praevia, are well seen by ultrasound, enabling elective caesarian section to be planned.

The evaluation of the fetus for congenital abnormalities is best performed at 16–18 weeks' gestation, at which time the major organs are visible on ultrasound. Neural tube abnormalities such as *anencephaly* and *spina bifida* (Fig. 143) can be detected.

Many genetic disorders such as *Down's syndrome* can also be detected around 16–18 weeks. Ultrasound may demonstrate structural abnormalities. Amniocentesis allows aspiration and subsequent analysis of the amniotic fluid. This is performed by passing a needle percutaneously under local anaesthesia into the amniotic fluid using ultrasound guidance.

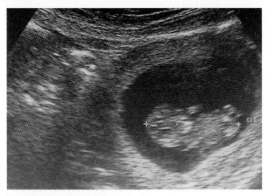

Fig. 142 Ultrasound of fetus.

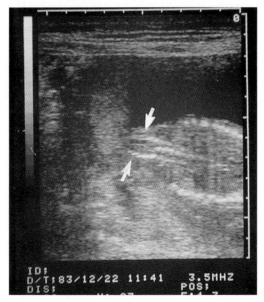

Fig. 143 Ultrasound showing spina bifida.

11 / Gynaecological imaging

Ultrasound   The uterus and ovaries are clearly seen on ultrasound when the bladder is full. Normal ovarian follicular cysts are small and disappear at ovulation. Pathological cysts are usually larger. Malignant cysts may have a solid component, whereas benign cysts are typically thin-walled; however, differentiation of benign from malignant cysts is not reliable on ultrasound alone.

CT and MRI   CT and MRI provide excellent visualisation of the pelvic organs and are useful in assessing the extent of spread of gynaecological malignancies (Fig. 144).

Contrast studies   Hysterosalpingography is used in the investigation of infertility. The uterine cervix is cannulated and contrast is injected to outline the uterine cavity and Fallopian tubes (Fig. 145). Normally, the tubes are patent bilaterally and of fine uniform diameter. There is free spill of contrast into the peritoneal cavity. Following pelvic inflammation or surgery, the tubes may be occluded, or adhesions around the fimbrial ends may prevent spillage of contrast. Tubal patency may be restored by balloon dilatation or by surgical means.

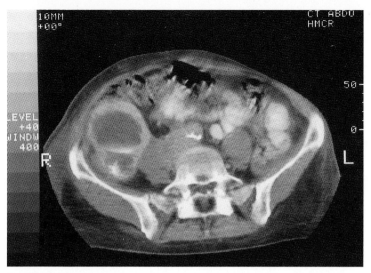

Fig. 144 CT of pelvic tumour.

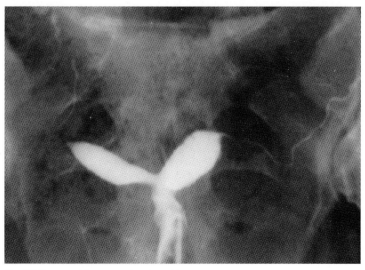

Fig. 145 Hysterosalpingogram showing a bicornuate uterus.

12 / Breast imaging

Mammography   The mortality from breast cancer can be reduced by early detection with mammography. The technique requires special low-kilovoltage equipment and meticulous attention to quality control. Drawbacks of a large-scale screening programme include the small risk of inducing breast cancer by radiation and the high level of expertise required to interpret the images. A national breast screening programme has been introduced in the UK for women aged 45–60.

In addition to screening, mammography is useful in the evaluation of palpable breast lumps (Fig. 146). Features suggesting carcinoma include a spiculated soft tissue density, microcalcification, distortion of the normal breast architecture and skin thickening (Fig. 147). Aspiration is frequently performed for cytological diagnosis.

Ultrasound   Ultrasound is particularly useful in the diagnosis of simple cysts of the breast in young women (Fig. 148) and avoids the risks of radiation. The ultrasound appearance is of a fluid-filled, thin-walled cyst with posterior acoustic enhancement. Aspiration of the cyst contents may be performed for diagnostic and therapeutic purposes.

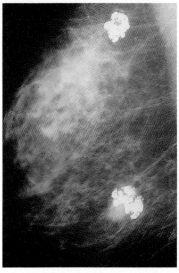

Fig. 146 Mammogram showing benign fibroadenomas.

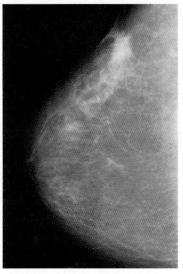

Fig. 147 Mammogram showing carcinoma.

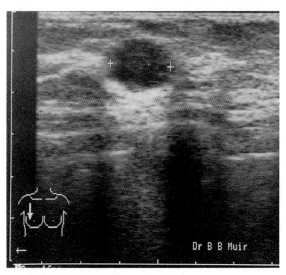

Fig. 148 Ultrasound showing simple breast cyst.

Index